HERBS FOR CANKER SORES AND MOUTH ULCERS

Soothing Remedies, Harnessing Wisdom To Relieve Nature's Bounty Through Effective Strategies

DR. JEREMY ALLEY

Disclaimer:

The information provided in this book, is intended for general informational purposes only and should not be considered as professional advice.

The author has made every effort to ensure the accuracy of the information presented. However, readers are advised to consult with a qualified healthcare professional before attempting any herbal remedies or making significant changes to their wellness routine. Individual health conditions vary, and what may be suitable for one person may not be appropriate for another.

It is important to note that the author is not in any endorsement deal, partnership, or affiliation with any organization, brand, or company mentioned in this book. Any references to specific products or services are based on the author's personal experience or general knowledge and do not imply an endorsement or promotion of those products or services.

Contents

Overview

Herbal treatments have long been valued for their inherent therapeutic abilities in the field of health and wellness. This book explores the intriguing realm of herbal remedies, with a particular emphasis on how well they work to treat mouth ulcers and canker sores. We must recognize the ancient knowledge that herbs provide in enhancing general health as we set out on this trip.

Greetings from the World of Herbal Medicines

Traditional medicine has always included herbal treatments, which are made from a variety of plants and botanical sources. This section delves into the extensive background and many uses of herbal remedies. Herbs have been used extensively in medicine to treat a wide range of conditions, from topical applications to tinctures and teas. It is necessary to comprehend the underlying theories of herbal treatments before delving into their possibilities for treating mouth ulcers and canker sores.

Knowing About Mouth Ulcers and Canker Sores

Mouth ulcers and canker sores can be painful and interfere with day-to-day activities. An extensive examination of the nature of various oral irritations is given in this part, which also covers possible triggers, symptoms, and causes. Gaining a thorough grasp of the causes of mouth ulcers and canker sores opens the door to investigating specific herbal remedies that deal with these problems at their core.

The Potency of Herbal Remedies

Herbal treatments have a special power since they frequently use the therapeutic qualities that plants naturally possess. This section of the book concentrates on particular herbs that are useful in treating and preventing mouth ulcers and canker sores. We examine the herbal companions that can offer relief and advance dental health, from chamomile to aloe vera. Knowing the science underlying these herbal remedies enables people to choose wisely when integrating natural methods into their daily wellness regimens.

It's important to approach the world of herbal remedies for mouth ulcers and canker sores with an open mind and a dedication to holistic well-being. People can explore a natural path toward oral health and find relief from the discomfort associated with these common disorders by fusing traditional wisdom with contemporary understanding.

CHAPTER ONE

ANATOMY OF MOUTH ULCERS AND CANKER SORES

Common oral disorders that can be painful and uncomfortable include mouth ulcers and canker sores. It is essential to comprehend the anatomy of these conditions to effectively manage and avoid them. Canker sores are small, superficial lesions that usually appear on the inside of the cheeks, lips, and tongue, among other soft tissues of the mouth. The term "mouth ulcers," which refers to a variety of oral lesions, can also impact the palate and gums.

How Do Canker Sores Occur?

Aphthous ulcers, sometimes referred to as canker sores in science, are excruciating oral sores. These lesions typically have an oval or spherical shape with a red border and a white or yellowish center. While the actual etiology of canker sores is yet unknown, certain meals, hormone fluctuations, and stress may all play a role in their development. Canker sores cannot be spread like cold sores, which are brought on by the herpes simplex virus.

Reasons And Initiators

Effective therapy and prevention of canker sores depend on an understanding of their underlying causes and triggers. Although the precise origin is unknown, several variables are thought to be involved, such as hormonal changes, oral trauma (e.g., biting the inside of the cheek), and deficits in vital minerals (e.g., zinc, iron, and vitamin B12). Other potential factors include underlying medical disorders like inflammatory bowel disease, citrus fruits and spicy foods, and emotional stress.

How To Spot Mouth Ulcers

There is a wider range of oral lesions that are not limited to mouth ulcers, and each has unique characteristics. They may appear as various forms of ulcers or as canker sores. It is essential to diagnose these ulcers to receive the right care. Common varieties include recurring aphthous stomatitis (canker sores), traumatic ulcers brought on by physical trauma, and viral ulcers linked to illnesses like herpes simplex. Furthermore, it is crucial to have a complete diagnosis because mouth ulcers may be a sign of underlying systemic disorders such as autoimmune diseases or nutritional deficiencies.

As we explore herbal treatments for mouth ulcers and canker sores, it's critical to understand the variety of these oral diseases and adjust our treatment strategies accordingly. Herbal medicines provide a comprehensive and natural substitute for conventional pharmaceutical interventions, regardless of the goal: symptom relief or prevention.

CHAPTER TWO

BASICS OF HERBAL REMEDIES

To begin using herbal medicines for mouth ulcers and canker sores, one must comprehend the basic ideas that underpin this type of treatment. Across many cultures, herbal treatments have been used for centuries to treat a wide range of health problems by utilizing the therapeutic qualities of plants. When it comes to mouth ulcers and canker sores, these treatments frequently concentrate on reducing pain, encouraging healing, and taking care of the underlying causes of these oral irritations.

Advantages Of Complementary Medicine

Herbs provide a holistic and all-natural way to treat mouth ulcers and canker sores. Herbal therapies are frequently well-tolerated by the body, in contrast to some conventional medications that may have negative effects. The pain and inflammation brought on by various oral disorders can be lessened by the anti-inflammatory, antibacterial, and calming qualities of several herbs. Herbal medicines may also improve oral health in general, offering advantages beyond short-term discomfort relief.

Selecting High-Quality Herbs

Proper herb selection is essential for successful herbal medicines.

Many plants have shown promise in the treatment of mouth ulcers and canker sores. Commonly used for their anti-inflammatory and therapeutic qualities include herbs including calendula, chamomile, licorice root, and aloe vera. To guarantee the efficacy and purity of your herbal treatments, make sure you select high-quality herbs from reliable suppliers.

Comprehending the distinct characteristics of every herb enables people to construct customized concoctions that cater to their requirements.

Making Herbal Decoctions And Infusions

Making herbal infusions and decoctions is an important part of using herbs to treat mouth ulcers and canker sores. Herbs are steeped in hot water to extract their therapeutic qualities in infusions while boiling herbs results in a more concentrated solution in decoctions.

For example, infusions of calendula and chamomile can be swished in the mouth as a calming rinse. Topically, licorice root infusions can be used to aid with healing.

Comprehending the suitable ways of preparation guarantees that people fully utilize the medicinal properties of the selected plants.

Exploring herbal therapies for mouth ulcers and canker sores requires a comprehensive grasp of the fundamentals, acknowledging the advantages of herbal healing, choosing herbs wisely, and becoming skilled in the preparation of potent infusions and decoctions. This all-natural method of maintaining dental health not only treats current issues but also enhances general health.

Herbs For Mouth Ulcers And Cancer

Mouth ulcers and canker sores can be excruciating, frequently making it impossible to eat and speak. Although several over-the-counter drugs can be used to relieve oral issues like these, herbal remedies offer a safe, natural option.

Calendula: The Antiseptic of Nature

Derived from marigold flowers, calendula has potent antibacterial qualities. It works well as a natural anti-inflammatory and antimicrobial treatment for mouth ulcers and canker sores. Calendula gel or ointment applied topically can alleviate pain by promoting healing and reducing inflammation.

Aloe Vera For Calm Comfort

Because of its calming qualities, aloe vera is a well-liked herbal treatment for several skin and mouth ailments, including canker sores. Aloe vera gel applied directly to the damaged region can help improve healing and ease pain. Its antibacterial and anti-inflammatory properties haveten the healing process.

The Calming Effect Of Chamomile

Because of its soothing and anti-inflammatory qualities, chamomile helps people with mouth ulcers and canker sores.

Applying a gel laced with chamomile or rinsing the mouth with chamomile tea can help ease pain and inflammation and facilitate a more comfortable healing process.

Sage For Dental Well-Being

Because of its astringent and antibacterial qualities, sage is useful in the treatment of mouth ulcers and canker sores. By reducing discomfort and preventing infection, gargling with sage tea or using mouthwash infused with sage can help maintain good oral health.

Root Licorice: An All-Natural Remedies

Because of its therapeutic qualities, licorice root has long been used. Glycyrrhizin, which has antiviral and anti-inflammatory properties, is present in it. Canker sores can heal more quickly and feel less painful if licorice root extract or gel is applied topically.

The Immune Boost Of Echinacea

Echinacea is well known for strengthening the immune system.

It can help treat canker sores in addition to being widely used to prevent colds and the flu. Drinking echinacea tea or supplements can strengthen the immune system and help the body fight against the root causes of mouth ulcers.

Additional Potent Herbs

There are a few other plants that may help with mouth ulcers and canker sores. Herbal remedies such as goldenseal, which has antibacterial qualities, and myrrh, which has calming benefits, are worth trying.

People might experiment with many herbal medicines to see which one works best for their particular problem.

Herbal treatments offer a holistic and all-natural way to treat mouth ulcers and canker sores. From immune-boosting qualities to antibacterial and anti-inflammatory qualities, each of the herbs listed has special advantages. By incorporating these herbs into dental care practices, you can help many common oral problems recover more quickly and reduce the discomfort they cause.

CHAPTER THREE

MAKING RINSES AND MOUTHWASHES WITH HERBS

Herbal medicines provide a safe and natural way to relieve the discomfort associated with mouth ulcers and canker sores. Herbal mouthwashes and rinses are a useful approach to including herbs in your dental hygiene regimen.

Homemade Herbal Toothpaste Recipes

You can customize the ingredients of your herbal mouthwash to suit your needs and tastes. Sage might be a useful addition because of its well-known antibacterial qualities. Steep dried sage leaves in hot water, filter, and let cool before using to make sage-infused mouthwash.

Another herb to think about is chamomile, which has anti-inflammatory properties. Making chamomile tea, allowing it to cool, then rinsing with it makes a chamomile mouthwash. These homemade mouthwash recipes offer a healthier substitute for store-bought mouthwashes.

How To Use Herbal Rinses Well

To get the most out of herbal rinses for mouth ulcers and canker sores, you have to utilize them skillfully. Before spitting it out, make sure the rinse has reached every part of your mouth by swishing it around for at least 30 seconds.

Repeating the procedure several times a day is recommended to maintain dental cleanliness and encourage healing, particularly after meals. Herbal rinses can help maintain a healthy environment for your oral tissues by lowering inflammation and inhibiting bacterial growth.

Using Herbs In Regular Dental Care

Incorporating herbs into your regular oral hygiene practice can help prevent and manage mouth ulcers and canker sores in addition to mouthwashes and rinses. Known for its calming qualities, aloe vera can be directly applied to afflicted regions. Herbs like echinacea or calendula used for toothpaste or mouth gel can also have long-term advantages.

The anti-inflammatory and antibacterial qualities of these herbs promote good dental health generally. Maintaining good oral hygiene and minimizing the recurrence of canker sores can be achieved with regular dental care regimens that use herbal components.

Herbal treatments provide a comprehensive and all-natural method of treating mouth ulcers and canker sores. Using custom-made mouthwashes, efficient rinses, or regular integration of herbs into dental hygiene regimens, these treatments offer a mild yet effective means of enhancing oral health and reducing discomfort.

CHAPTER FOUR

MEDICATION ADVICE FOR GUM HEALTH

It is important to take care of your teeth, and you may prevent and treat mouth ulcers and canker sores by adopting particular dietary practices. A healthy, well-balanced diet is essential for promoting the body's inherent healing mechanisms.

Items To Steer Clear Of

Mouth ulcers and canker sores can hurt more when certain foods are consumed. Citrus fruits, tomatoes, and chili peppers are examples of foods that are acidic and spicy and can irritate delicate oral tissues, increasing pain and delaying healing. Avoiding crunchy and rough meals like chips and crackers can also help stop additional aggravation.

Fruit juices and sodas are examples of highly acidic or sugary drinks that should be avoided since they might impede the healing process and cause canker sores. Hot foods and drinks should be avoided since they might exacerbate the pain and suffering that come with mouth ulcers.

Vitamins For Remedy

By including particular nutrients in your diet, you can speed up healing and lessen the incidence of mouth ulcers and canker sores. Vitamin C is essential for immune system performance and tissue healing. It is typically found in citrus fruits, strawberries, and leafy greens. Foods high in zinc, such as nuts, seeds, and legumes, promote wound healing and maintain dental health.

The health of the mucosal membranes in the mouth depends on the B-complex vitamins, which include folate and B12. Rich sources of these vitamins include meat, fish, dairy products, and leafy greens. Consuming foods high in probiotics, such as yogurt and fermented veggies, can help improve dental health by encouraging a stable and balanced oral microbiota.

Hydration And Its Effects

Staying well hydrated is essential for good health in general and for preserving dental health and avoiding canker sores in particular.

Water keeps the mouth wet, encourages salivation, and aids in the removal of toxins, all of which can worsen ulcers.

It's important to stay hydrated throughout the day, especially after eating acidic or sugary foods that can irritate your mouth.

Herbal teas that don't have any added sugar or acidic ingredients can be a calming substitute. It's best to limit your intake of alcoholic and caffeinated drinks since they can exacerbate oral irritation and cause dehydration.

Key dietary strategies for treating and preventing mouth ulcers and canker sores include eating a balanced diet, avoiding trigger foods, adding healing nutrients, and drinking enough of water. These procedures assist the body's natural healing processes and improve dental health in general.

CHAPTER FIVE

WAYS OF LIVING CHANGES FOR PREVENTION

Because canker sores and mouth ulcers can be uncomfortable and unpleasant, people look for effective treatments and preventative measures. Although there are several traditional therapies available, adopting lifestyle modifications can be quite important in averting the development of these oral annoyances.

Stress Reduction

Stress is one important component that leads to the development of canker sores. Elevated stress levels have the potential to compromise immunological function, increasing susceptibility to oral health problems. By using stress-reduction methods like yoga, deep breathing exercises, or meditation, people might lessen their stress levels and possibly cut down on the frequency of canker sores.

Habits Of Oral Hygiene

Keeping your mouth as clean as possible is essential to managing and avoiding canker sores. Frequent, good brushing and flossing will help get rid of bacteria and lower your chance of getting infections that might cause mouth ulcers. The risk of developing a canker sore can be decreased by using a toothbrush with soft bristles and avoiding toothpaste with abrasive ingredients.

The Impact Of Lifestyle Decisions On Dental Health

Certain lifestyle decisions can have a direct effect on oral health, influencing the likelihood of mouth ulcers and canker sores. For instance, it is well-recognized that excessive alcohol intake and tobacco usage can exacerbate oral health problems. In addition to improving general health, giving up smoking and consuming alcohol in moderation can also help create a healthier oral environment, which lowers the risk of unpleasant mouth sores.

Another lifestyle decision that might improve dental health is eating a diet high in vitamins and minerals. The health of the oral tissues depends on consuming enough iron, zinc, vitamin B12, and folate. These vital nutrients can be obtained from eating a range of fruits, vegetables, and whole grains, which may help prevent canker sores.

Intentional lifestyle modifications can be a proactive strategy for mouth ulcer and canker sore prevention and management.

The frequency and severity of these oral annoyances can be greatly decreased by individuals through stress management, good mouth hygiene, and conscientious lifestyle choices.

CHAPTER SIX

SUCCESS STORIES AND CASE STUDIES

Experiences from everyday living provide important information on how well herbal treatments work for mouth ulcers and canker sores. Examine case studies that describe people's experiences utilizing herbal remedies, including their achievements and setbacks.

Viewed through the eyes of those who have experienced alleviation, have a fuller comprehension of the real-world application of these therapies.

Actual Herbal Medicine Experiences

Testimonials include personal stories from people who have included herbal treatments in their dental hygiene regimens. Learn about the various ways that herbal remedies have helped people manage and avoid canker sores and mouth ulcers via personal stories.

Those looking for natural solutions to their dental health issues can find inspiration in these stories.

Our goal in providing you with extensive information regarding herbal treatments for mouth ulcers and canker sores is to empower you.

The information provided here is a great starting point for anyone looking to improve their oral health, whether they are investigating these options as a preventive strategy or as a means of treating current problems.

CHAPTER SEVEN

INTEGRATING HERBAL AND MODERN METHODS

Mouth ulcers and canker sores can hurt, making it difficult to eat and talk comfortably. While there are many therapies available in modern medicine, a comprehensive answer may be achieved by fusing modern methods with ancient herbal remedies.

Combining Conventional And Modern Medical Practices

Combining conventional herbal therapies with contemporary medicine can provide a more thorough course of treatment for mouth ulcers and canker sores.

For millennia, several civilizations have utilized conventional herbal remedies to ease mouth discomfort. These treatments frequently concentrate on lowering inflammation, encouraging healing, and easing discomfort.

Aloe vera, which has anti-inflammatory and wound-healing qualities, is one traditional treatment.

Aloe vera gel applied directly to the injured region can help reduce pain and hasten the healing process. Another plant with anti-inflammatory qualities that can be used as a mouthwash to reduce pain and support dental health is chamomile.

Another option is licorice root, which has antiviral and anti-inflammatory qualities and is prized in traditional medicine. Mouth ulcers may heal faster and with less inflammation if licorice root paste or gel is applied to the damaged area. Moreover, mouth rinses that fight bacteria and promote dental hygiene can be made using the antibacterial qualities of some herbs, such as thyme and sage.

Even while using traditional herbal medicines might be beneficial, it's important to incorporate them within a larger treatment plan that also makes use of contemporary medical techniques. Benzocaine or hydrogen peroxide-containing over-the-counter topical gels or mouthwashes may offer immediate pain relief and infection protection. It is essential to speak with a healthcare provider to make sure that the herbal remedies you have chosen don't conflict with any prescription drugs and to get specific guidance on how to treat mouth ulcers.

Collaborating With Medical Professionals

Seeking advice from medical experts is essential to properly managing mouth ulcers and canker sores. In addition to recommending suitable therapies, dentists, oral surgeons, or general practitioners can provide insightful information on the underlying causes of oral ulcers.

It is imperative to notify healthcare experts about the selected herbal treatments when combining them with contemporary methods to guarantee a safe and well-coordinated approach.

Medical personnel can evaluate therapy progress, provide advice on dosage, and provide information about possible drug interactions.

To stop recurring mouth ulcers, they could also recommend dietary adjustments, lifestyle adjustments, or stress-reduction techniques. Frequent dental examinations can also improve oral health in general and help identify any underlying problems early on.

A comprehensive approach to treating mouth ulcers and canker sores involves fusing conventional herbal medicines with contemporary medical techniques.

Combining these methods under the supervision of medical experts guarantees a comprehensive and individualized treatment plan that takes into account the root causes and symptoms of mouth ulcers.

Aloe Vera: The Natural Healing Gel

Because of its calming qualities, aloe vera is a useful herbal treatment for mouth ulcers and canker sores. Aloe vera plant gel is extracted, and its antibacterial and anti-inflammatory qualities may aid in pain relief and healing. Relief and a quicker recovery can be obtained by directly applying a small amount of aloe vera gel to the affected area.

Licorice Root: An Anti-Inflammatory Agent Found In Nature

Traditional medicine has utilized licorice root due to its anti-inflammatory qualities. Licorice root contains a chemical called glycyrrhizin, which may have anti-inflammatory properties and help lessen the pain and discomfort of canker sores. An effective treatment for mouth ulcers is to make a mouthwash out of licorice root by steeping the root in hot water.

Chamomile: Relieving Tension

Another herbal medicine that can be used to treat canker sores is chamomile, which has mild and calming effects. Once at room temperature, chamomile tea can be used as a mouthwash to reduce soreness and inflammation. Chamomile's potential efficacy in promoting oral health is attributed to its antioxidant and anti-inflammatory components.

Echinacea: Increasing Immune Function

Echinacea is well known for strengthening the immune system. Its capacity to strengthen the immune system may help canker sores and mouth ulcers heal, even though it is frequently used to stop or shorten colds. Taking echinacea tea or supplements can be viewed as a comprehensive strategy to assist the body's inherent healing processes.

FINAL VERDICT

Examining herbal treatments for mouth ulcers and canker sores can provide a holistic and all-natural method of treating oral discomfort. Herbs with the ability to reduce inflammation, ease pain, and aid in the body's healing processes include echinacea, aloe vera, licorice root, and chamomile. It is important to consider personal sensitivities when using these cures and to seek the counsel of healthcare specialists.

Summary Of Herbal Remedies

In summary, licorice root's anti-inflammatory qualities, chamomile's calming benefits, echinacea's immune-boosting qualities, and aloe vera's soothing gel offer potential herbal remedies for canker sores and mouth ulcers. By including these treatments in one's dental hygiene regimen, discomfort may be relieved and a quicker recovery may result. Nonetheless, one must proceed cautiously when using herbal medicines, taking into account personal allergies or sensitivities. Seeking advice from medical experts guarantees an informed and customized strategy for treating mouth discomfort.

Taking Control Of Yourself Via Knowledge

When people are equipped with information regarding herbal remedies for oral health issues, they can make well-informed decisions regarding their health. By being aware of the characteristics and possible advantages of herbs, people can investigate all-natural options for treating mouth ulcers and canker sores. People can actively participate in their dental health and general well-being by being informed and taking into account both conventional wisdom and scientific facts.